101 Things I Wish I'd Known When I Started Using Hypnosis

Dabney Ewin, MD, FACS

Crown House Publishing Ltd
www.crownhouse.co.uk
www.crownhousepublishing.com

First published by
Crown House Publishing Ltd
Crown Building, Bancyfelin, Carmarthen,
Wales, SA33 5ND, UK
www.crownhouse.co.uk

Crown House Publishing Company, LLC
PO Box 2223
Williston, VT 05495, USA
www.crownhousepublishing.com

British Library of Cataloging-in-Publication Data
A catalogue entry for this book is available
from the British Library.

13-digit ISBN 978-184590291-9
10-digit ISBN 184590291-2
LCCN 2009936271

The history of hypnosis is littered with stories of the downfall of practitioners who were lured into grandiosity by the siren song of cures that border on the miraculous. I dedicate this composition to my wise and precious wife, Marilyn, who has been my anchor to keep my feet on the ground while my head was in the sky.

Contents

i

Foreword

I asked Dr. Ewin to tell me in one word how he would describe the essence of his professional life as a physician. His answer was clear, quick and passionate. This is a man whom we all admire for his intelligence, his effectiveness in treating patients, and his teaching. Yet it comes down to one word, his word: enthusiasm.

The words and phrases that come to a physician working over a lifetime are guides to the art of therapy. In many patients, symptoms fall into the cracks between mind and body and this elusive interface can only be reached with scientific insight and intuitive understanding. Dr. Ewin understands this and emboldens his art with vigor.

Dr. Ewin "believes his patients can get well, because they do." With his words, images and suggestions, noted throughout this little book of wisdom, he changes the way his patients think, feel, and behave. He knows the mind can change the way the brain functions and he also knows the brain can change the way the mind functions. In hypnosis, he makes this healing resonance between mind and body happen again and again. Simply put, his patients become whole again.

I encourage each reader of this wonderful book to embrace Dr. Ewin's lifetime of experience, make it fit into your own style, and teach it to others as you travel the path of your own career.

For these are the secrets, these are the keys, and these are answers that work.

Peter B. Bloom, MD, Clinical Professor of Psychiatry,
University of Pennsylvania School of Medicine,
Past President, International Society of Hypnosis

Preface

Always read the *little* book.

Charles Dunlap, MD

One day in medical school our pathology professor, Dr. Dunlap, rolled in a small library of about thirty books, resembling the *Encyclopedia Britannica*. He told us it was a monumental compilation of everything that was known about diabetes, published in 1920, before the discovery of insulin. Then he held up a book of about 200 pages, and said, "This was published in 1930, *after* the discovery of insulin. *Always read the little book.*"

In addition to the economy of time, my experience has been that a small book is likely to be a clear message by a knowledgeable author. My copy of *The Pursuit of Simplicity* by Edward Teller, PhD, the physicist who produced the hydrogen bomb, is 167 pages. Sometimes a large edited book is a collection of little books (chapters), but that is rare.

I have sought to make this publication as *little* as possible, consistent with the message. Over the years I have jotted down various insights about hypnosis to pass on to my students, and this is the result.

Malek's Law: *Any simple idea will be worded in the most complicated way.*

Every violation of Malek's Law is a victory for education and communication. At the risk of being overly elemental, I have sought to reverse this common phenomenon, so that the most complicated idea is presented in the simplest way.

Dabney M. Ewin, MD, FACS

Words

We are treating people with words, so the dictionary and thesaurus are our pharmacopoeias. What we say, what we omit, and how we say it matters very much. Even without hypnosis, this is ancient knowledge. George Baglivi (1704), a prominent seventeenth century Italian physician wrote: "I can scarce express what influence the physician's *words* have upon the patient's life, and how much they sway the fancy; for a physician who has his tongue well hung, and is master of the art of persuading, fastens ... such a virtue upon his remedies and raises the faith and hope of the patient ... that sometimes he masters difficult diseases with the silliest remedies (emphasis mine)." (Duct tape for warts? If you can influence the patient to believe it, it works!) What we call placebo in the waking state is much enhanced in hypnosis.

1. Seems

This is a very helpful word when doing a regression to a traumatic incident, particularly if there was a perceived danger of death.

I can say "Even though it *seems* like you might be killed, isn't it nice to know that it only *seems* that way, because we already know that you're going to survive this, no matter how bad it *seems*."

2. Yet

This is a good word to use when doing analysis.

Ideomotor signals are unconscious body movements initiated by an idea, like nodding the head when agreeing, and are generally referred to as body language. In hypnosis we use finger movements.

When setting up ideomotor signals, I have a finger to signal "I'm not ready to answer that question *yet*," or "I don't want to answer it." He/she may not want to ever answer it, but when that finger rises I say to the patient "That's all right, you don't have to answer it *yet*, but you will know when the time is right to understand yourself fully." A question the patient doesn't want to answer is surely an important one, and we don't want the finality of just signaling, "I don't want to answer."

3. Stop (not quit)

Quitters are losers.

In our society, to quit school is a disaster, to quit a job causes wonder if you were about to be fired and to quit a marriage is a failure of commitment and sad for the kids.

Quit has negative emotional content built into the word. When the whistle blows at 5 o'clock, we *stop* work, but don't quit. It's emotionally much easier to stop a bad habit than to quit it.

4. Give up

Give up is a synonym for surrender.

Any boy who's ever wrestled with a bully who had him in a neck lock knows the humiliating demand "Do you give up?" If the pain is so bad that he gives up, there is residual anger and resentment.

Winston Churchill inspired the whole free world during the Second World War with his words "We will never surrender!" A therapist who tells a patient/client to *give up* a bad habit should consider giving up using that phrase. It's better to *abandon, discontinue, reject, refuse,* and so on.

5. Try

The word implies failure.

I only use it when I *don't* want something to happen. Sometimes it's fun to say "Try to keep from laughing" when I'm going to inject some local anesthetic. They usually laugh, even though it hurts some.

Picture yourself in the dental chair, and the dentist says "Try to relax." Trying takes effort; relaxing is the opposite. How much better to just say "Relax."

The Nike advert doesn't say "Try harder" – it says "Just do it."

6. Feel

The subconscious is the feeling mind, and the conscious is the logical one. Many feelings cannot be described as logical.

When using ideomotor signals in hypnoanalysis, I ask if it *feels* "yes" or *feels* "no." The conscious veridical facts are not the problem; it's what the patient *feels* is true that causes symptoms.

7. Sense

This calls more for an intuition than a feeling. It's a subtle difference.

When I'm asking about Cheek's seven common causes of symptoms (conflict, organ language, motivation, past experience, identification, self-punishment and suggestion (COMPISS), I ask "Do you *sense* that you are being affected by a conflict?" It's different from asking "Do you feel …?" because they may not have any feeling one way or another about this new idea.

8. Bother

People are afraid of pain, but they don't mind a little discomfort as long as it doesn't cause pain.

When I'm going to draw blood, as a waking suggestion I say "You may feel a little pressure, but it won't bother you." This is a negative suggestion (Thing 21), so of course it does bother them a little, but at least it didn't hurt. They've been instructed to interpret what they feel as pressure, and that doesn't bother them very much.

9. Normal

The word I use whenever
I can't think of anything specific
to suggest as a goal.

Between diarrhea and constipation,
obese and emaciated, hyperimmune
and immunodeficient, there is a wide
field of comfort that we all agree is
normal and good.

10. Fix

Sounds like a good word, but no man wants to hear it if he remembers what happened when he was a boy and his folks took his dog to the veterinarian to be "fixed."

All gamblers know how to bet when "the fix" is in. It's better to *repair* or *revise.*

11. Burn

This word is one of the descriptors of pain.

When we say "It burns" we're describing a particular type of pain. So I avoid using it when treating a burned patient. I say "Notice how the *involved area* is becoming cool and comfortable," not the "burned area" is comfortable, which is like saying "Try to relax" (Thing 5).

12. Problem

This is the right search word to Google the subconscious mind of a patient with a psychosomatic disorder.

My opening comment to a new patient is "Tell me about your *problem*." This is very different from "What's the matter with you?" or "How can I help?" which will be answered with a list of headaches, indigestion, insomnia, and so on.

The *problem* is emotional, and the answer will give a clue. Sometimes it's a volunteered negative, for example "It's certainly not fear," which of course means that suppressing fear is what is on the mind. There may be a Freudian slip or a gratuitous clause that hints at the emotional problem.

13. Daydream (vs. imagination)

When I'm asked to imagine something, I simply daydream about it. I cannot distinguish between daydreaming and imagining, but there seems to be a subconscious difference for many patients. They may have been told "You're imagining things," or "It's all in your imagination." I find that adults feel more in control of their daydreams than their imaginations, and when I want to do some imagery I ask them to simply daydream it.

On the other hand, some children have been admonished to "Stop daydreaming and get busy with your homework," so imagining is a better word for them than daydreaming.

I like Sarbin's (2006) definition: "Hypnosis is believed-in imagination." My experience has been that anyone who can either imagine or daydream can experience hypnotic phenomena. The goal of all our training is to learn how to present it so the patient does indeed believe it.

14. Precious

Precious is the best single word I
know for ego strengthening, along with
"You're just as good as anybody else, and
you don't have to prove that to anybody.
It's all right to just be yourself."

We so easily forget that we are
created precious (not perfect) and we
can find meaning in our lives.

15. Safe

A sense of safety is missing from the life of everyone who is anxious. Toward the end of my induction of a patient who is anxious, reluctant, or uncomfortable, I don't hesitate to say "You're safe here, and I won't let anything happen to you. It's all right to go as deep as you need to go to solve this problem."

One definition of anxiety is that it is a chronic state of fear, and an unending problem for an anxious person is the feeling that "I have to be on guard to protect myself." What a relief to be told in trance that you can suspend that feeling for a little while, and be *safe*, because I will protect you. It builds rapport.

Smoking Cessation

Since the report of the Surgeon General in 1964, and subsequent passage of many restrictive laws, cigarette smoking in the United States has fallen from near 50 percent to a fairly unvarying 21 percent of "incorrigible" smokers. The hypnosis literature is full of reports claiming high rates of success, but with only short term, verbal follow up. I give them little credence because smokers often lie to their doctors to avoid being reprimanded. Very few people resume smoking after a year of abstinence, and I hope we will see a prospective controlled study with chemical follow-up at one year.

16. Quit.

Telling a patient "You have to quit smoking" has two fatal errors. We live in a free country, and we rebel against being told that we *have to* do anything. It took almost fifteen years for us to accept being told we have to wear seat belts, when common sense and factual data say it may save our own lives.

It's un-American to be a *quitter*, and we resist it emotionally (Thing 3). When a patient seeks help I say "You *need* to *stop* smoking," and he/she can readily accept that as good advice, not an intrusion on choice, and not a call to the ignominy of being a quitter.

17. I'm a smoker

When a patient tells me
that the problem is "I'm a smoker,"
it's like saying the problem is that
"I'm an Eskimo."

It implies that it's an unchangeable fact of life and treatment will be futile. That idea is unacceptable, and I reframe it immediately to "Isn't it more true to say that you are a *human being* who chose to learn how to smoke?" When that change is accepted, we can get to the issues of how, when, and why he/she chose to *learn* to smoke, and see if a new choice is the way to solve the problem.

18. Ex-smoker

I've heard discussions about telling a patient to become an ex-smoker. I don't care for the idea of being an ex-anything. Who wants to be an ex-convict, ex-communist, or an ex-beauty queen?

I tell my smoking patients that the goal is to become *normal* again. It's *normal* to breathe air, and it's so abnormal to inhale smoke that the only living creature that doesn't run from smoke is the human, who had to learn how to do it.

19. Non-smoker

Who wants to be a nonentity, or a non-Nazi, or a non-terrorist?

Again, if the goal is to characterize the patient, let it be to become *normal* again.

20. Lapse (instead of relapse)

Relapse implies that we are back where we started, and nothing of value has happened.

If a smoking patient has abstained for a month, and then lights up a few cigarettes, I don't treat it as a failure, just a *lapse* in the ongoing success.

All through school we take a vacation every summer, and it's just a lapse in our ongoing education. In September we don't start again in first grade – we move ahead to the next year's class.

I point out that "Every success leads to more success, and if you can succeed for a month, you can do it for two, then four, and eight, and so on."

21. Negative suggestions

Negative suggestions often backfire.

If I tell you "Don't think of an elephant," the first thing you must do is think of an elephant, so you'll know what not to think about.

So we can predict what will happen when someone says to a person in a long leg cast, "Don't pay attention if it starts to itch, because you can't scratch it."

How many times have I heard a nurse tell a child "This won't hurt," just before giving an injection that is routinely followed by a scream. The suggestion that "You will *not* feel like smoking anymore" is a sure loser.

22. Impossible

Impossible is a word that turns a negative suggestion into a positive one.

Instead of saying "You won't want to smoke," I can say *"Let it be impossible to* put a cigarette in your mouth without first looking at it, and making a conscious choice about protecting your lungs."

23. Addiction

This word has lost its meaning in scientific communication, and I generally seek to avoid it. It no longer refers to a bodily need for a particular chemical, and is used indiscriminately to describe strong emotional desires such as being *addicted* to chocolate, sex, sports, and now foreign oil.

The patient who thinks of him/herself as an addict has adopted a fixed idea that he/she is helpless to overcome the problem. This is particularly true with incorrigible smokers (about 21 percent of the US population).

Granted nicotine is a powerful drug, but if a person can wake up and fix a cup of coffee before the first cigarette, it was not a chemical deficit that woke him/ her up. The only patients that I put on patches are the rare ones who light up before they get from the bed to the bathroom in the morning. For the others, I point out that the problem is *not* a chemical addiction, it is a craving, and it can be changed.

24. Induction on first visit

It only takes five minutes to do a simple eye roll induction and give a suggestion that "The next time you are ready to go into trance, you will find it very easy to quickly go twice as deep as you are now." A patient who comes for hypnosis is prepared for it, and even if he/she doesn't think anything trancelike happened, will return for the next visit somehow wondering if he/she really will go twice as deep.

For those concerned about hypnotizability, remember that hypnotizability is a stable trait and can be measured at any later time, or the Hypnotic Induction Profile (HIP) can be used as the first induction and simultaneously measures hypnotizability.

I treat smoking patients for three visits, and if the first visit is just a detailed history taking or hypnotizability testing, they did not get the hypnosis they came for, and leave disappointed and smoking as before. At a meeting in Europe I heard a report of a carefully controlled smoking study complete with tests of hypnotizability. No induction was done on the first visit. One third of the subjects deserted, and did not return to participate after the first visit. The doctors blamed it on a lack of motivation on the part of the patients, but I think the failure to do an induction on the first visit was a flaw in the design of the study.

25. Three issues maintain smoking behavior

One of Aesop's fables tells of a village with a prize for the strong young man who can break a bundle of sticks. After all the other contestants have failed, the village idiot unties the bundle and breaks the sticks one at a time to win the prize.

I think there are three "sticks" in the smoking bundle, and I endeavor to break them one at a time:

i.   **The concept that it has social value** (subconscious fixed idea – see Thing 60). All of us who formerly smoked can recall coughing and turning green as we learned to inhale, but we persevered because we believed it had value: the older guys who smoked got all the girls, or you were a sissy if you didn't smoke, or all the beautiful movie actresses smoked, and so on. We know that *if you violate a fixed idea it causes anxiety* (Thing 60). I set out to remove this idea first and foremost, usually with a regression. *It is the paramount issue* for the incorrigible smoker. I have friends who can determinedly (left brain) give up smoking for the forty days of Lent, endure forty days of anxiety, and on Easter Saturday light up and say "It calms my nerves."

ii.   **Nicotine** has a chemical effect that I think is much less addictive than is generally believed. Patients who put on nicotine replacement patches frequently still experience the anxiety of violating a fixed idea (Thing 93); and some even secretly smoke while wearing the patch. After adrenalin, nicotine is the strongest known stimulant drug, and it's an oxymoron to say "I take a stimulant to calm my nerves." What calms the nerves is accommodating to the fixed idea. Once I've identified and removed the fixed idea, I have the patient switch to regular Carlton's (almost nicotine free) for a week, smoking all he/she wants, but reading the Surgeon General's warning before each cigarette. This removes nearly all of the nicotine from the body, and stopping smoking does not cause much chemical repercussion. It's interesting that in their study of 12,000 smokers Tindle et al. (2006) noted that people who smoke "light" (low nicotine) cigarettes are more than 50 percent *less* likely to stop smoking than those who smoke regular cigarettes. That finding is incompatible with chemical addiction.

iii. **Habit** change is easy with hypnosis. On the third visit I make a personal self-hypnosis tape reviewing the fact that the fixed idea has outlived its usefulness, that breathing air is normal, and that my patient will be pleased and proud of his/her accomplishment. Since I don't get to do chemical tests at one year, I do not have factual data on my quit rate, but believe I get over 50 percent with incorrigible smokers (Ewin 1977).

26. Smokers lie to their doctors

Smokers lie to their doctors just like alcoholics do.

The British Thoracic Society study (1983) of 1,500 patients coming to clinic for the treatment of smoking related diseases did plasma thiocyanate and carboxyhemoglobin tests at one year.

These tests showed that only 10 percent of these "highly motivated" patients had stopped smoking, and 26 percent who said they had stopped had elevated thiocyanate and carboxyhemoglobin levels consistent with continued smoking.

Hypnosis was not tested in this study – only doctor's advice with and without booklet material, nicotine gum, and placebo. We will only have *believable* evidence-based statistics on the value of hypnosis for smoking cessation when someone does chemical studies at one year.

Pain

In the emergency room, a skilled hypnotist can use the frightened patient's spontaneous trance to get rapid relief of *acute* pain, control bleeding, reduce a fracture, and allay fear. The office-based hypnotist is most likely to deal with *chronic* pain. Inflammatory processes are a common cause of chronic pain. Pain is an integral part of inflammation, so in these cases anti-inflammatory suggestions of being cool and comfortable are indicated. When the diagnosis is psychogenic pain, we must remember Milton Erickson's dictum "The symptom is a solution." Muscle spasm pain is severe and often psychogenic, and once mechanical and chemical causes have been ruled out, our duty is to help find a better solution.

27. I must believe in what I'm saying to the patient

A patient in trance picks up insincerity and uncertainty like it was on radar, and it causes loss of trust and rapport. Sometimes I have to parse my words literally in order for me to *believe* what I want to say.

With chronic pain patients, I insinuate into my induction "We all know that no pain lasts forever." By assuming that a dead person does not experience pain, I can rationalize that if my treatment doesn't work (which happens at times), and the patient ultimately dies still having pain, it literally won't last forever.

I once said this to a disabled patient during a demonstration, and she came out of trance crying, and hugged me and exclaimed "Nobody ever said that to me!"

✳ 28. You will have all the comfort you need

This is a good positive suggestion that does not mention the word pain.

Also, it doesn't say there will be no pain at all, and it raises the question of how much comfort suffices. I learned this from the warm and gentle Bertha Rodger, MD, anesthesiologist, and past president of ASCH.

29. Tolerable

Tolerable is a good word to use when seeking to lessen pain on the 0–10 scale.

If the patient is at 8, "Would it be all right to lower the intensity of the pain to a tolerable level?" With an ideomotor "yes," then "Would 7 be *tolerable* for you?" "No," then 6, 5, 4, 3 (progressively lowering the numbers to an ideomotor "yes").

Tolerable is an attitude, not a number, and I've had patients who could function OK at 5, which would be quite intolerable for me.

30. Once everything that can be done, and should be done, has been done, pain has no value

There's an obvious right time to
say this during therapy.

I learned it from Kay Thompson.
I point out to my patients that pain is
nature's valuable alarm system.

If I put my hand on a hot stove, the pain is an
immediate warning that if I don't do something
I will get tissue damage. But once I remove my
hand, any pain I feel has no further value, and
needs to be turned off.

31. Inflammatory pain

Celsus gave us the four cardinal signs of inflammation in 45 AD: calor, *dolor*, rubor, and tumor (heat, *pain*, redness, and swelling). The patient is aware of the heat and pain (subjective), and the doctor can see the redness and swelling (objective).

The anti-inflammatory suggestion only needs to address the subjective component, so "Let the involved area become cool and comfortable" suffices.

The suffix "itis" in a diagnosis indicates an inflammatory disorder (e.g. arthritis, vasculitis, bursitis, spondylitis, cellulitis, bronchitis). Many of these respond to specific therapies – a steroid injection into an inflamed bursa or colchicine for acute gouty arthritis – and they should be treated accordingly. Nonetheless, nearly any inflammatory pain syndrome can be improved with hypnotic stress relief and direct suggestion to be cool and comfortable. This is particularly true with burns. Only the *initial* burn pain is from the heat injury, but the longtime *background* pain is inflammatory.

32. Constant pain

Constant pain is nearly always psychological in my experience. Almost any physical pain can be *temporarily* relieved by medication, rest, sleep, or positioning.

When a patient says the pain "never goes away" even in sleep, or "it's always there," I listen for "I live with it." That is a subconscious equating of pain with life, and just as one cannot be without life for five minutes, he can't be without the pain for five minutes.

The intake history will include three things happening simultaneously (Ewin's triad): (1) a life threatening incident with fear of death; (2) mental disorientation (helplessness) from concussion, drugs, anesthesia, and so on; and (3) pain. At a subconscious level, as long as the pain is there he can't be dead yet! I have written on the Constant Pain Syndrome and the hypnotic technique for relief (Ewin 1980, 1987).

33. Muscle spasm pain

Muscle spasm pain can be very severe. In a good trance with muscular relaxation, it will clear temporarily, but often recurs out of trance.

John Prussack, MD has a marvelous video of a man with severe torticollis that fully relaxes in trance and recurs immediately on alerting with a count up technique. Finally, he gives the suggestion "When your subconscious mind knows that you can keep your neck muscles as comfortably relaxed as they are right now, you will open your eyes and come back fully alert." The choice is to get well or stay in trance forever. It worked, and I now use that double bind alerting suggestion for patients with muscle spasm pain.

One common muscle spasm pain is "night cramps" in the legs and feet, usually in older persons. I believe it has to do with the acetylcholine release that normally occurs during sleep. It is relieved by waking up and walking the floor. It's off-label, but I learned a long time ago that 25 mg of over-the-counter Benadryl will relieve it in 5–10 minutes without waking up and walking.

Techniques

When I started my surgical training, the first book my mentor recommended was entitled *Surgical Errors and Safeguards*. We do not need to repeat the errors that have been made in the past. *Primum non nocere*, first of all, do no harm. Good technique comes from our own experiences and from listening to those who have "been there and done that." There are things to avoid and there is what to say, when to say it, and how to say it. Hypnosis is an empathetic involvement with another, and as we interact with our patients/clients, we evolve in our tone of voice, choice of words, what we emphasize, and our timing.

34. Full bladder

Alexander Levitan (in a personal communication) points out that we should never start an induction if either the patient or the therapist needs to urinate.

Our earliest training in civilized life is "Don't wet your pants." This is powerfully embedded in the subconscious mind, and as the bladder fills it will progressively interfere with the other subconscious work being done in trance.

35. Inductions

There are many techniques for the induction of hypnosis. What do they have in common?

It seems to me that all of them tend to turn off left brain conscious logic and encourage a *shift into daydreaming* (good or bad imaginings, or emotional states).

The goal becomes dissociation from conscious logic, an "altered state of consciousness" with focused attention, and in which a subject lowers critical testing and is more open to suggestions. Even though hypnotizability has measurable characteristics of a trait, and direct suggestion works best for those who have this trait, the ability to go into a state of trance sufficient to *analyze* implicit imprints with ideomotor signals seems to be almost universal.

- *Confusion* of the conscious mind is relieved by just turning it off. Milton Erickson could rapidly induce an eyes open trance with his confusion techniques.

- *Eye fixation* with an upward gaze tires the weak levator palpebrae muscles so that the eyes ultimately close from fatigue, and the illogical idea that they are closing because the hypnotist suggests it is an abandonment of conscious logic.

- *Eye roll* induction is unique. With eyes closed and eyeballs rolled upward, it is almost impossible to think of a mathematical problem or anything logical. For me, it rapidly brings on a meditative state where my mind can be blank (left brain turned off), or I can do ideomotor self-analysis or analyze my own dreams.

- *Repetitive meaningless stimuli* like a swinging watch, a blinking light (particularly if timed with alpha waves), or a military drum beat require no logical thought or attention, and lead into trance-like states requiring no logical thinking. Counting sheep to turn off the day and get to sleep is amusing, but historically it works. Monotonous verbal repetition acts the same. Dull lectures induce daydreams, and the best time to pass the plate in church is right after the sermon, when we either feel inspired by the message or guilty for dozing off.

- *Back drop* induction is used often by stage hypnotists because it is almost instantaneous. Asking the subject to "Imagine that your body is a board, standing on end" has the compliant volunteer in an instant daydream, with left brain logic turned off.

- *Trauma.* The first law of nature is self-preservation. When there is a perception that life is threatened, nothing else matters. Fear is the strongest of all emotions. We have fire drills because in an emergency we immediately drop logic and go into automatic, and a pre-programmed escape plan avoids desperate measures like jumping out of a tenth story window.

36. First induction double bind

I don't like to argue with a patient about whether or not he/she was hypnotized.

I start my first induction with a question. "Do you know what you are most likely to do that will interfere with this?" "No." "You're likely to *try* too hard. Or you may try to be the best patient I ever had. I want you *not* to give a hoot whether or not you do it right, and I *want* you to avoid any attempt to test it because you have to be out of trance to test whether you are in. So just do what I ask you to do and let it happen" (Thing 5).

If the patient subsequently protests that he/she wasn't hypnotized, I agree. The only way he/she would know is to be focused on that issue and testing. So I say "Of course not. You were testing, which I told you interferes with success. Next time, you can see what happens when you don't give a hoot, and just do what I ask you to do. On the other hand, there's nothing wrong with getting well without *ever* going into trance, except that it takes a lot longer and I make more money."

37. Intake question is like a Google – ask the wrong search word, and get a useless answer

On the same day, I Googled "anesthesia" (American spelling) and got 10,900,000 references, then used "anaesthesia" (British spelling) and got 3,080,000 references.

In trance, patients tend to assign very literal meanings to the words that describe the way they picture their lives. This has led me to devise a carefully worded intake history that evokes maximal clues to the patient's subconscious content. The wording is on page 25 of Ewin and Eimer (2006).

38. The patient's name carries emotion

I ask a new patient "What do you *like* your *friends* to call you? May I call you that?" I'm expecting to ask some intimate questions, and this is an indirect suggestion that I want to be thought of as a friend, and to have permission to enter the circle of friendship. I'm amazed at how many people don't like their given names, and don't even like some nicknames that their "friends" call them.

Pronunciation matters. I did a demonstration in England with a doctor named Kathleen, who preferred the English form with the accent on the first syllable. I inadvertently used the Irish form, with the accent on the last syllable, and I could *feel* the loss of rapport even though I didn't realize what I had done until later. The IRA was bombing England at the time, and my demonstration bummed out also.

39. Importance of the last question on the intake

The last question of my intake is "Is there anything else you think I ought to know?" Invariably, if the patient answers it, he/she is telling me the problem.

It's as though the subconscious is saying "Since you never asked the right question, I'll *tell* you what the problem is." If the answer is "No," I hope I took good notes, because the patient feels he/she has already told me what's important, even if it was just in a gratuitous clause.

40. One issue at a time

Patients often have multiple complaints,
sometimes even bringing in a written list.

In doing hypnoanalysis, when this occurs I ask "If
you could solve *one* problem today, what would it
be?" The answer is what's on top of the patient's
mind, and it's what we should concentrate on.

Often, it's not what seems most important
to me, but as we unravel it some of the other issues
usually fall into place or lose some of
their importance.

41. Piloerection test

Every hair cell has a tiny muscle called a piloerector. It's what makes a cat's hair stand up when it "bristles" in defense.

When I do an intake on a new patient, if the hair on the back of my neck stands up, I won't hypnotize that patient. It means that I don't like him/her, and I think it's best for us both if I refer that patient to another therapist.

42. Value of marathon treatment

Helen Watkins taught us the value of this intense form of hypnotherapy. As a new patient gives the intake history, all sorts of subconscious memories, associations, and feelings are being scanned and are fresh. Continuing with therapy at this time is much more productive than weekly visits.

My outcomes are regularly better and use less time when I set up four to six consecutive hours with a patient. Strike while the iron is hot! At the least, I schedule my initial visit for two hours, and make sure to include an induction (Thing 24) with some ego strengthening suggestions.

43. Return to actual date from an age regression

When a patient is in a true regression and abreacting in the present tense, the suggestion "Come back to today" may not end it because *today* is the day he/she has regressed to, and confusion results.

One should be specific and say something like "Time now to return to today, November 12, 2009, here in my office and feeling safe and secure."

44. Amnesia is a test for analgesia

When a patient goes deep enough to have the numbers disappear as he counts backward, he is deep enough to take a suggestion to produce analgesia sufficient to suture a laceration, relocate a dislocation, or manipulate a fracture.

Involuntary muscle spasm fights against fracture reduction, and the relaxation obtained with hypnosis makes it easy. I usually inject some local anesthetic into the hematoma of a Colles' fracture of the wrist, since it makes *me* feel more comfortable.

45. Make the subconscious issue conscious

Prescribe the symptom. *"Try* to have the tic."
This gets the benefit of the word *try* (see Thing 6) and what previously was an unconscious motor activity now becomes a conscious issue, except that it seems silly to consciously do it.

I have a couple of patients who are denizens of the French Quarter. They worry that they will not be able to get into the Mardi Gras costumes they have made so carefully. They come in early December, fearful of gaining weight during the holidays. I tell them to go ahead and enjoy the parties and even gain a little weight, and return on January 2 and we can get the weight controlled. Surprisingly, they've usually lost one to three pounds on the next visit, subconsciously controlling their intake without effort, and not feeling deprived.

46. Let the patient do his own brainwash

Fred Evans (1989) reported an interesting technique he literally called a "brainwash." I have gotten good, quick results using this with patients who come in with a long list of bizarre symptoms.

I say something like "You sound like you have accumulated so much crap in your brain that you can't sort it out. Why don't we do a brainwash and start off with a clean slate?" Then, in trance, the patient pictures a zipper around his/her head, we unzip and open the skull, and there is this awful, ugly, dirty brain. I gently take it out and place it in a bucket of lukewarm water, hose out the base of the skull until it's glistening clean, and then go to the bucket. I used to be ever so gentle, knowing as I do how delicate the brain is. I would use a soft sponge and mild detergent, and perhaps a cotton swab in the gyri to get it clean, then return it to the skull and zip it closed. Then we would pick *one* problem that really mattered and work on that (Thing 40).

Then I learned something. A patient told me I didn't know anything about really cleaning up, and his result was poor. So I said "Teach me how to do it right," and took him back and let him do the cleaning. He took a wire brush, some strong detergent, and hot water and really did a (daydream) number on his brain. He was tired of all the crap. I just shut up while he was focused on this, and asked for a nod of his head when he was through scrubbing. The clean brain was replaced, and the scalp zipped shut. It worked fine and he made a nice recovery. Since then, I have always let the patient do the cleanup.

47. Laughter enhances immunity

The autoimmune disorders (lupus, rheumatoid arthritis, psoriasis, etc.) are the most difficult chronic diseases we treat in medicine. Stress is implicated as part of the origin of most, and removing it often produces remission. The medicines that suppress immune function are powerful and usually have dangerous side effects. We need a healthy immune system to protect us from infections.

Specific stress reduction can be done by hypnoanalysis, but there is a universal non-specific remedy that is too often overlooked – laughter. Norman Cousins cured himself of ankylosing spondylitis with humor and the stress vitamin, vitamin C. His little book *The Anatomy of an Illness* (Cousins 1979) should be required reading for everyone in the healing professions. We benefit when we get serious about humor.

48. Laughing place

In hypnotic imagery it is common to seek a "safe place," a "special place," or even a "happy place." All of these are somewhat protective, internal, and self-soothing. Laughing is more a shared activity and gets us out of ourselves. A real smile starts in the eyes (looking outward), and projects an altruistic feeling of warmth – what we feel when we smile at a pet, a child, or a loved one.

For many years I have obtained good results directing my burned patients to go to their *laughing place* while I do all the work. In the Disney movie *Song of the South*, Br'er Rabbit sings "Everybody's got a laughing place." He was "born and bred" in the brier patch, a place where nothing can bother, nothing can disturb.

49. Use patient's own words

This is the left brain title under a right brain picture (Thing 58). If he says he stammers, for him it's different from stuttering, even though I consider them synonymous. If he says he "upchucks," I don't ask about vomiting or throwing up. If his headaches are "whoppers," I don't try to redefine them as migraines. I ask how often he has a whopper and what brings on a whopper. For him, migraines are something other people have.

50. You pray for me, and I'll pray for you

This has been a valuable strategy for me when treating religious patients who tell me they pray every day to get well. Nothing has happened after many prayers and the patient is in my office for treatment.

When I pray for myself, my subconscious mind starts rationalizing God's possible reasons not to grant my wish, because of any number of transgressions. But when I pray for someone else I have no negative feedback, and feel every expectation that something good will happen. So I suggest that we do something different, saying something like "God works in many ways. Would you be willing to approach Him in a different way, and instead of praying for yourself, ask God to give *me* the knowledge, understanding, and wisdom to be the means by which He heals you? I will pray for you, and you can pray for me."

I have to be careful with this, because it's like plugging into Louisiana Power and Light. It's powerful, and I must be *completely* trustworthy (godlike?). I take this seriously and do include the patient in my prayers, which makes that patient special. Perhaps I ruminate more deeply about the nature of the suffering of these patients. Sometimes the results are seemingly "miraculous."

51. If something bothers me, my patient will become disturbed too

Sir William Osler of Johns Hopkins, known as the father of medicine in the US, said "in the physician or surgeon no quality takes rank with imperturbability ... it means coolness and presence of mind under all circumstances, calmness amid storm, clearness of judgment in moments of grave peril, immobility, impassiveness, ... phlegm" (Osler 1905).

I have a noisy office on street level, and I have learned to include in my induction the positive suggestion "Paying attention *only* to the sound of my voice. Any other sound that you hear will be very pleasant in the background, and just help you to go deeper and deeper. It's comforting to know that the rest of the world is going on about its business, while you and I go about ours."

Some of my deepest trances occurred when they were putting up a building across the street. The pile driver made a loud "wham" and shook the building with every blow. My response was "Every time the hammer hits, it will drive you deeper and deeper," and I could use the time for therapy without spending time on deepening.

52. Finger signals make a patient more aware of true feelings

Awareness means "conscious of." Part of emotional illness is to suppress true feelings, and often a patient is unaware or unwilling to admit to them.

When I get an ideomotor response, I give a tactile feedback (I touch the finger and gently push it back down) and also give verbal feedback "That's right, the answer is …" It may surprise a patient to admit to an implicit negative or positive feeling that had been unknown or deemed unacceptable at a conscious level. But it is comforting because it is honest, and can be dealt with honestly. "And ye shall know the truth, and the truth shall make you free" (John 8:32).

53. Always add an endpoint

Always add an endpoint to a suggestion that would cause a problem if it continued indefinitely. Analgesia should last only "until it's healed" or post-op "as long as you need it."

I was asked to see a patient with a broken neck who had been in traction for six weeks and had bony healing, but could not sit up in a neck brace. Every time she sat up she got excruciating pain and had to lie back down immediately. Reviewing her treatment in trance revealed that on admission, when she was put in cervical traction the orthopedic resident had told her "Whatever you do, don't take off this traction and sit up, because you could be paralyzed for life." She was in a traumatic hypnoidal state at the time, and took it literally like a post-hypnotic suggestion. All I had to do was add an endpoint by saying "It was a good idea at the time, but now that it's healed it is safe to sit up comfortably." If the resident had added an endpoint such as "Don't sit up *until we tell you to,*" there would have been no problem.

54. Pre-hospitalization suggestion

In a hospital all kinds of things are said that have unintended consequences. I may go to the recovery room and hear a nurse saying "Wake up Mr. Jones, *it's all over.*" If he's frightened and interprets that pessimistically (see Thing 64), it's not what he should hear. I go and tell that patient "Joe, this is Dr. Ewin. Your operation is *completed* and you're OK." We must be precise in our language.

Alexander Levitan, MD taught me to suggest "If anybody says anything that's less than helpful, let it be as though they said it in Chinese (or any language they don't understand), and it will have no effect at all."

I gave this suggestion pre-operatively to a member of my family who had a simple release of a DeQuervain's tenosynovitis of the wrist, and the anesthetist had said "My uncle had that operation, and they ended up having to amputate his thumb." Fortunately, she just smiled and immediately translated the comment into unintelligible Chinese.

It's a common thing for people (called "Job's comforters") to think it's reassuring to say "You sure are lucky … (you didn't get killed, lose a leg, etc.)." It doesn't make anyone feel lucky – it simply implants an additional catastrophic thought at a time when the patient most needs reassurance. It should be heard in Chinese.

A negative expectation (nocebo) tends to be accepted without testing (instinctive self-protection), and it trumps a placebo, which first requires some education for positive expectation to be accepted (Colloca et al. 2008).

55. A specific question often acts as an indirect suggestion

There is danger of implanting a false memory with a leading question.

Martin Orne demonstrated this in the BBC documentary on hypnosis (Orne 1982).

All questions in hypnosis should be open and non-specific:
"What's happening?"
"And then …?" and so on.

56. Avoid delayed response to a suggestion by using a broad alerting suggestion

Delayed response is a well documented phenomenon, and is one of the dangers of not removing undesirable suggestions given during trance. The lack of an *immediate* response to a post-hypnotic suggestion does not mean that it had no effect. André Weitzenhoffer (1957) reports in his book the case of a student who took the Stanford Scale test with no apparent effect but woke up the next morning with a partial paralysis. I have a published letter to the Editor of the *American Journal of Clinical Hypnosis* describing three cases of delayed effects (Ewin 1989). This has led me to an all encompassing *wipeout* alerting suggestion, saying "When I say three, you will open your eyes and come back fully alert, sound in mind, sound in body, and in control of your feelings. One (pause), rousing up slowly, two (pause), *three.*" An increase in tone and volume on "three" helps effect a change to full alertness. Richard Kluft (2007) has stressed the importance of fully terminating trance, and the dangers of neglecting it.

My premise is that if the patient is suggestible enough to accept one suggestion in trance, he/she is also suggestible enough to be sound in mind (not goofy), sound in body (no unwanted motor or sensory aberration), and in control of feelings (not an emotional disaster).

Miscellaneous Pearls of Wisdom

In medical school we used to classify keen insights and clever or astute discernments as "Pearls of Wisdom," or just Pearls. Sometimes they were simply philosophical thoughts, and often they could not be easily classified, but were worthy of recollection. In this section I have included some random observations, insights, and thoughts that have impinged on my experiences in life as a doctor who uses hypnotic concepts in daily practice. Perhaps this section should just be labeled "Pearls."

57. Nobel Prize for left–right brain function

Roger Sperry, PhD won the 1981 Nobel Prize for his studies of the difference in function of the two cerebral hemispheres. *Clinical experience* demonstrates that in a good trance the left brain functions are progressively shut down. Speech is a left brain function, and a subject in trance will not ordinarily *initiate* speech (but will answer and talk when so instructed), ordinary logic is abandoned in favor of trance logic, timekeeping sense is lost, and the analytical step-by-step sense is switched to global, metaphoric, and intuitive (right brain) processing of information.

Doing clinical work, I have found this knowledge very helpful in my understanding of what is going on with my patients as I do nonverbal (right brain) ideomotor questioning. Since most left brain functions are learned, children don't have a lot to turn off. They are simply not yet completely on, and children live easily in daydream and trancelike states. Animals function as though they have two right brains.

We must of course be aware that hypnosis is much more than Sperry's studies show, and that respected scientists disagree vigorously on details of its true nature. Nonetheless, it is a simple concept for me as a clinician working with a patient. I can drive a car without understanding all the machinery and electronics, and I can treat nearly all of the patients who come to my office. Sometimes a car has to be referred to a mechanic, and sometimes a patient must be referred to a more knowledgeable doctor.

58. Left and right are a title and a picture

Sperry's studies indicate that the left brain processes information in words, and the right brain processes the same incoming information in the senses (mainly sight, sound, and action – NLP anyone?).

The right brain visualizes the information, and the left brain puts a verbal descriptive title under it. David Pedersen, MD, of Oxford, theorizes that in trance, with the patient's left brain function inhibited, the voice of the hypnotist becomes the substitute for the verbal input of the left brain to the right brain (Pedersen 1994). He stresses how useful this concept is in clinical work, and I agree.

59. Dissociation requires association

In psychology, the word dissociation was always difficult for me to understand, because no one ever said what the patient was dissociating *from*. You can't dissociate without being first associated with something. When it became clear that left brain functions are shut down when a person is dissociated, I was able to make sense of the word.

60. Fixed idea
(*idée fixe* of Pierre Janet)

Anyone carrying out a post-hypnotic suggestion or an imprint has his/her behavior unshakably determined by the fixed idea. A fixed idea can be violated but only at the expense of experiencing anxiety.

Phobias are fixed ideas and locating their origin by a regression in hypnosis allows reframing to a better idea.

61. Strong emotion makes one vulnerable to waking suggestion

I had a patient with a hysterical paralysis who had lost the tip of his finger in an industrial accident. He was very upset because he was not a laborer; he was just working a part time job before beginning teaching music at a local university. The skin closure was tight and the orthopedist said "Don't bend your finger, because you will pull out the stitches."

Three months after the stitches were removed he was still unable to bend the finger. In a regression to the surgery I learned what the surgeon said, removed the suggestion, and pointed out that the sutures were already out and the wound healed. He rapidly regained a full range of motion. An emotional state focuses like a trance and a statement at that time can act like a post-hypnotic suggestion.

The strong emotion at the time of a death-bed wish affects the recipient like a post-hypnotic suggestion. It becomes a fixed idea and may be carried out at considerable inconvenience. In his famous poem "The Cremation of Sam McGee," the poet Robert Service (1940) says "A promise made is a debt unpaid," and it's a long story as he is determined to carry out his friend's dying request (Thing 62, Law iv).

In therapy, we know that if you can put an idea in, you can remove it. Correct diagnosis requires that we identify the suggestion we want to remove. A regression to the incident and reframing that it was a good idea at the time, but it has now outlived its usefulness, will resolve a problem that started at a time of high emotion.

62. Coué's Laws

Emile Coué was a French pharmacist who studied hypnosis in Nancy under Liébeault around 1900. He is considered the father of auto hypnosis, and gave us the classic self-suggestion "Every day, in every way, I'm getting better and better." He also gave us five laws that have stood the test of time:

i.   **Law of Reversed Effort (or Effect).** *If a person fears that he cannot do something, the harder he* tries, *the less he is able.* In fact, he tends to do the opposite of what he wishes to do. I've seen this many times with insomnia, with excellent students who are failing exams, and with impotence. They all solve themselves naturally if one doesn't *try* too hard.

ii. **Law of Dominant Effect.** *When the will* (I translate as left brain) *and the imagination* (I translate as right brain) *are at odds, the imagination invariably wins.* I see this in nearly every phobia that I treat. If someone imagines that it is very dangerous in an elevator, even though his left brain logic says it's not, he will walk up ten flights of steps to avoid the elevator.

iii. **Law of Concentrated Attention.** *An idea tends to realize itself, within the limits of possibility.* Choices in daily life tend to favor the realization of the idea. I recall reading that as a boy Jimmy Carter dreamed of becoming President. He sought and obtained an appointment to Annapolis and became the only member of his family to have a college education. Then he went into politics, was Governor of Georgia, and ran as an almost unknown candidate for President, and won. His idea realized itself.

iv. **Law of Auxiliary Emotion.** *The intensity of a suggestion is proportional to the emotion that accompanies it.* An idea goes into the subconscious with very little force if there is no emotion attached. When there is strong emotion, particularly terror, an idea is strongly fixed in the subconscious. Henry Beecher, MD at Harvard, studied placebos and found that the greater the stress, the more effective the placebo (Beecher 1956).

v. **Law of Autosuggestion.** *A suggestion only produces the condition to be transformed into an autosuggestion, that is to say* accepted *by the deepest self. The same incidents produce different effects depending on the subject who receives the suggestion.* In other words, all suggestion is self-suggestion and a subject still has a choice to accept (self-suggest) or reject a new idea. This is why it is wise when doing ideomotor work to ask "Is it all right … (to regress to birth, to visit the White Light, to stop smoking now, etc.)?" A "yes" answer means the patient is open to accept what is contemplated, and a "no" means I may as well drop the subject for now, because nothing is going to happen.

Coué maintained that he had never cured anyone: "I teach you a method, and you can cure yourself."

63. Law of Pessimistic Interpretation

David Cheek said "If a statement can be interpreted optimistically or pessimistically, a *frightened* person will interpret it pessimistically." This is protection against perceived danger. An antelope that sees the bushes wiggling and (pessimistically) moves away for fear it is a lion is more likely to survive (natural selection) than one that assumes it's a wart hog and keeps on grazing. In a "haunted house" a squeaking sound could be a rusty door closing or it could be a ghost. If you're already frightened, it's a ghost! Many of our patients arrive frightened about their health and are inclined to interpret any imprecise statement pessimistically.

When President Reagan was shot through the lung I saw a news item in the *Los Angeles Times* stating that the surgical resident said "This is it!" Reagan blanched, and unable to talk (he was intubated), he scribbled a note to the nurse "What does he mean, *this is it?*"

Pity the poor frightened patient whose doctor's advice was "You have to learn to live with it." If he takes that literally (pessimistically), the only way to be without it is to die. I spend a good part of my therapy time removing that suggestion and replacing it with "There's nothing wrong with living *without* it." We must use precise language to avoid pessimistic interpretation by a frightened patient.

64. Law of Perceived Reality

If a patient believes something to be true, it is true for him/her. We know that in any kind of forensic work the veridical facts are what matter, and external corroboration is needed before we accept information obtained in trance. Not so in clinical work. Regardless of the reality, if a patient believes something to be true, he/she will think, feel, and act as though it were true. We need to meet the patient where he/she is, or lose rapport. If we treat an idea with respect, even though we don't agree, we put ourselves in a position to lead.

In treating psychosomatic disorders, I often ask a patient to regress to the *first time* this symptom was too important, and occasionally (rarely) he/she arrives at a past life. When this occurs, it is usually associated with the (supposed?) cause of death in the past life – a tomahawk to the head, a sword in the stomach, a suffocation, and so on. I interpret that as a protective idea (a sort of trance logic) that as long as the symptom is there, "I can't be dead yet." If I get an ideomotor confirmation that this thought is occurring, I can point out in trance that it really doesn't matter anymore, because we know that you *did* die in that life, and you are back now in a new life. "Do you really still need this symptom to prove that you're alive now, in a new body, at a new time, and in a new place?" An ideomotor "No" answer makes it easy to say "In that case, since you don't need it anymore, would it be all right to just let it go and get on comfortably in this new life?" I have no idea if the patient had a previous life, but I can treat a patient who believes he/she did have one by accepting the fact that it *is* true for that patient.

65. Laws of Hypnotic Depth

A patient tends to go as deep as he/she needs to go to solve a problem. A patient tends to stay as light as necessary to protect him/her self.

Just my personal observation, so it's Ewin's Law.

66. "Dreams are the royal road to the unconscious"

"Dreams are the royal road to the unconscious" (Freud 1900).

I perceive imagination (*daydreams*) as key to hypnosis and would rewrite it as "*Hypnosis* is the royal road to the unconscious." Freud started with hypnosis but gave it up early in his career. He apparently was not good at inductions and was dissatisfied with his results using only direct suggestions (Kline 1966).

67. First three years of life

The importance of the first three years of life in personality development is well documented. Regressions to preverbal memories are of inestimable value in hypnoanalysis. Even though it is rarely possible to validate what the patient expresses, it is therapeutic to treat it as real (Thing 64) because it comes from the patient. If the patient believes that it's true, it *is* true for him/her, and reframing an early trauma (real or imagined) is often curative.

Childish reasoning thinks like the rooster Chanticleer. He noted that the sun rose after he crowed, and concluded that it rose *because* he crowed.

68. Anamnesis

Anamnesis is the correct word for what we call *history*. Mnesis is memory; amnesia is no (verbal or explicit) memory. Anamnesis is what the patient did not forget or repress, so it's all the patient can give us from *explicit* memory. The verbal "history" contains Freudian slips, non-responsive answers to questions, sighs, volunteered negatives, and gratuitous or qualifying clauses that come from *implicit* memory, and guide us to the subconscious mind set. What is repressed is seminal in psychosomatic medicine, so we must *listen in literal.*

We learned from the polygraph (lie detector) that a sigh negates what was just said. A volunteered negative expresses what the patient is guarding against, so a volunteered "It's not caused by fear" means that it *is* caused by fear. When I ask a pre-op patient "How do you feel about this operation?" and get "OK (pause), I guess," the qualifying "I guess" tells me he subconsciously lied, saying "OK," then felt guilty for lying and added "I guess" to clear his conscience. I need to find out what reservations he has about the procedure before I operate.

69. Self-analysis using pendulum or ideomotor signals

Nobody taught me that I could analyze my own symptoms by using self-hypnosis and setting up ideomotor finger signals or by using a Chevreul pendulum in the waking state. It works well for me to analyze my own dreams at the time I become aware of the dream. What is the affect – fear, anger, love, guilt, sadness, etc.? What happened yesterday to trigger it? Who is in it – me, spouse, parent, sibling, God, enemy, etc.? Does it refer back to something in my past? If so, before 30, or 20, or 10, or 5, etc.? Would it be all right to bring it up to a conscious level? And "Voila!" there it is. All of these need to be "yes" or "no" questions.

Triggers for dreams are interesting. I recall an awful nightmare I had, in which there were six bodies laid out and I stabbed each of them in the heart. I woke up horrified, then used the above technique to interpret the dream. It turned out that in the course of my surgical career I had had six cardiac arrests, with varying outcomes, but always of deep concern to me at the time. I learned whatever lesson there was to learn from each, and did not think about

them consciously. I wondered what had triggered
this dream, which occurred while I was on my
vacation. What came up was that I was at a friend's
home and had stumbled upon a book of stories I had
enjoyed as a child. The author was Bret *Harte*.
Words activate old memories, functioning like search
words to Google the subconscious.

70. Self-regression

Part of self-analysis includes age regression. I was able to validate a self-regression to the fourteenth day of my life from the microfilm records of the hospital where I was born. I reported it in the *American Journal of Clinical Hypnosis* (Ewin 1994).

71. The symptom is a solution

One of Milton Erickson's most profound observations!

We all know that halitosis is better than no breath at all.

In the movie *Forrest Gump*, the little crippled boy was being hounded by the bullies and felt terrified and helpless, with no solution. Jenny shouted "Run, Forrest, run." He did, and escaped, and from then on he had a "solution" that was really a disabling symptom – whenever he was stressed, he would run – finally all the way across the United States.

72. Target organ

A chain is as weak as its weakest link, and a body under stress gets symptoms first in its target organ (weakest link).

We experience our emotions in our bodies. Over and over again I have done regressions to the *first time* the problem occurred, and found that the target organ was selected when a highly emotional incident occurred, associated with a trauma or illness involving that organ. Even when the careful medical evaluation is normal, recurring headaches may occur under stress in a patient whose introduction to life was the painful head squeezing of a forceps delivery, or a recurring cough in a survivor of childhood whooping cough, or diarrhea in a survivor of typhoid fever.

73. Trance logic

With ordinary (left brain) logic turned off, the hypnotized mind is open to uncritically accepting clearly irrational and paradoxical situations or statements.

In New Orleans during the big drive against illiteracy, the advertising companies got some of the federal money and we had large billboards saying "Learn to Read." Louisiana advertises itself as a "Dream State."

74. Pygmy in the land of giants

This analogy was used by William J. Bryan, Jr., MD to describe the dilemma of an abused child.

A pygmy in the land of giants has to believe that the giants know where they're stepping or go crazy, being constantly alert to protect himself. Some abused children do go crazy but those who don't tend to grow up subconsciously believing "there must be something wrong with me" or the giants (who know what they're doing) wouldn't have treated me that way.

It's imagined guilt and in trance it can be treated by calling on reality testing to recognize that the adults were sick, not the child, and it has to be left behind. When we change an idea, we change an illness.

75. Migraines and hypoglycemia

Migraine headaches frequently respond poorly to hypnotic suggestions for pain relief. I have found that many of my migraineurs also have functional hypoglycemia, which Hans Selye (1946) showed is the end result of chronic stress (Thing 86). A five hour glucose tolerance test will confirm it. Their dietary enemies are refined sugar, refined flour, alcohol, and caffeine.

I get good relief by putting these patients on a six feeding, low sugar, low refined carbohydrate, no alcohol, and no caffeine diet combined with hypnoanalytic sessions for general stress relief.

76. Shingles and vitamin B

Shingles is an infection of the ramus of a nerve by the virus (herpes simplex) that causes chickenpox, resulting in an inflammation of the sensory nerve and dermatitis in the skin area served by it. In healthy young people it heals in four to six weeks, but in the elderly it frequently fails to heal and becomes a chronic painful post-herpetic neuralgia.

Since vitamin B complex deficiency *causes* a polyneuritis (beriberi), it seems reasonable to me that we must make sure there is no B deficiency when trying to heal a neuritis. Combining hypnotic suggestions for pain relief with high doses of B complex and B12 injections, most of my patients have recovered in less than four weeks without getting a post-herpetic neuralgia. I am unable to find any controlled studies of B complex in the literature on shingles, and recognize that this is using "armchair" logic. Nonetheless, it works for post-herpetic neuralgia, and I don't know if it's the hypnosis or the vitamins or the combination that does it.

77. Warts and warm, cool, or tingle

Warts are a viral infection and when treated with
cautery, freezing, surgery, topical salicylates, interferon
injections, and so on, about 30 percent keep recurring.
Traditional treatment is OK, but when warts are on
the bottom of the foot, under the nails, on the genitalia,
or on the vocal cords, hypnosis is the treatment of
choice. When cured with hypnosis they almost never
recur, presumably because the patient's own immune
system has effected the cure. With children, direct
suggestion of cure usually suffices. With post-pubertal
teens and adults, I frequently have to use ideomotor
signals and go through Cheek's seven common causes
of symptoms (Thing 7) to remove any emotional
inhibition to healing. Surprisingly, about half of these
patients have sexual issues that inhibit healing, and
once dealt with they heal easily.

I used to suggest that the area of skin around the
wart would get warm, with more blood supply
bringing in antibodies and so on, but often that didn't
work. When it didn't, the patient would give an
ideomotor signal that cold would have been easier. I
now ask the patient's subconscious to choose from

four choices — make it warm, cool, tingle, or a way of your own. When the patient gives his/her ideomotor choice in trance, I touch the wart (obviously not with venereal warts) for a tactile feedback, and have the patient daydream the change. When I get an ideomotor signal that the change has occurred, I say "Keep it that way *until it's healed* (Thing 54). Your body knows how to heal, and you can turn this over to your body and give it no more conscious attention."

I avoid adding self-hypnosis because all of the experimental studies that have included it have had miserable statistical results. In their controlled, prospective study that included self-hypnosis, Felt et al. (1998) got only a 5 percent cure rate, and I wrote an editorial on my opinion of why the results did not exceed even placebo response (Ewin 1998). I get an 80 percent cure rate doing analysis and specifically avoiding self-hypnosis (Ewin 1992).

78. Get treated yourself

One of the best things that happened to me was to be successfully treated with hypnosis early in my study of the subject. It convinced me of the validity of this form of treatment and gave me a strong sense of conviction that my patients could solve their problems too, if I gave them choices.

Emile Coué said "Conviction is as necessary to the *suggester* as the subject. It is this conviction, this faith, which enables him to obtain results when all other means have failed (emphasis mine)."

Luke Skywalker: "I don't believe it."
Yoda: "That's why you fail."
The Empire Strikes Back

Dr. A. A. Mason, who reported the only known cure of a case of the "incurable" congenital ichthyosis of Brocq (1952), told us that he mistakenly thought the patient was covered with warts and *confidently* gave the suggestions to heal. Later, when biopsies showed that it was "incurable," he was unable to heal any of eight subsequent patients who had the same disorder (Mason 2007).

Scripture says "For if the trumpet give an uncertain sound, who shall prepare himself to the battle? So likewise ye, except ye utter by the tongue words easy to be understood, how shall it be known what is spoken? For ye shall speak into the air" (1 Corinthians 14:8–9).

79. "The best doctors are Dr. Diet, Dr. Quiet, and Dr. Merryman" – Jonathan Swift

This threesome is worth remembering. Each is noted in the Bible.

- **Diets** in our time are often deficient. Vitamin C is our stress vitamin, and only guinea pigs, anthropoid apes, and humans have an inborn error of metabolism and don't make their own. Most of my hypnosis patients are in treatment because of various stresses, and the 60 mg/day (one glass of orange juice) RDA *recommended* daily allowance is not *optimal*; 60 mg is only enough to prevent scurvy, a fatal disease. I advise a multivitamin supplement plus 1,000 mg of vitamin C daily for my patients, and believe it helps, particularly because most of them are not eating a well rounded diet with lots of citrus fruit and uncooked vegetables, and are unlikely to change their eating habits significantly. Also, several studies show that a person who has one or two drinks per day has fewer heart attacks than one who doesn't drink at all. Scripture says "use a little wine for thy stomach's sake, and thine often infirmities" (1 Timothy 5:23).

- **Quiet** even for a few moments relaxes both physical and mental tension. Ernest Rossi's (1991) recognition of our daily ultradian rhythms, and the value of a short retreat at those times of day, has become part of my own self-care (I have a reclining chair in my office) and I recommend it to my patients. A few moments of feeling love or gratitude restores cardiac coherence (Servan-Schreiber 2004). "Be still, and know that I am God" (Psalm 46:10).

- **Laughter** is its own reward and controlled studies show that it enhances the immune system. Anecdotally, Norman Cousins' self-cure of the autoimmune disorder ankylosing spondylitis with laughter and vitamin C is classic (Cousins 1979). "A merry heart works like a medicine" according to Solomon (Proverbs 17:22).

80. Laughter therapy

A group in Shanghai uses laughter as prophylaxis against cancer. They were shown on the Noetic Science video series *The Heart of Healing* (1992). This fits with the anti-stress treatment that Norman Cousins used.

Pain and depression go together, and patients with either seldom laugh. Robert Heath, MD, Professor of Psychiatry and Neurology at Tulane, did experiments using deep probes into animal and human brains to locate a "pleasure center" in the septal region. In the booklet that summarizes his work (Heath, 1996) he says: "Physical pain of various origins was alleviated promptly and dramatically by electrical stimulation of sites in the brain's pleasure system. The pain of metastatic carcinoma, uncontrolled by high doses of morphine, for example, was relieved for as long as a week after stimulation of the septal region for 15 minutes (100 Hz, 3-5 amperes)" (Peacock, 1954). For seven months before she died, patient A-6 (L.W.) who had carcinoma of the uterus, received electrical stimulation of the septal region at intervals of one day to one week (depending on control of pain). During that period, she was essentially free of pain and required no further analgesic medication. He notes that *when pleasure takes over, pain disappears.*

I teach my patients to use self-hypnosis to find their "laughing place." In the Disney movie *Song of the South,* Br'er Rabbit sings "Everybody's got a laughing place" (Thing 48).

81. Hearing under anesthesia

Timid animals (rabbits, deer, humans, etc.) need to be aware of predators while there is still time for escape. They protect themselves with all five senses. But in order to close the eyes and sleep when danger lurks, they must depend on smell, taste, touch, and hearing. Of these, only hearing warns of danger before it is too late, and this is the last sense to go before actually dying.

We know how a mother with a newborn child can sleep through a thunderstorm, but becomes wide awake if the infant barely whimpers. This is selective hearing and can happen under general anesthesia, usually selecting the voices of the two people who are in control, the anesthetist and the surgeon.

The ultimate experiment on hearing under anesthesia was Levinson's test of anesthetizing a cat down to a flat line EEG, then bringing a dog into the lab. When the dog barked, the cat's EEG spiked (Levinson 1990).

When a patient's symptoms have been "Ever since my ... surgery," hypnosis with multiple ideomotor reviews will often recover something alarming that the surgeon or anesthetist said during anesthesia. The hypnotic technique to recover this is precise. None of those who say it can't be recovered have used David Cheek's technique (Cheek 1959, Ewin 1990). What is recalled has three qualities: (1) it is salient, (2) it is said by the surgeon or the anesthetist, and (3) it is said at an appropriate time during the procedure. At the time the initial incision is being made for an *exploratory* abdominal operation, the suggestion "Everything is OK" is inappropriate, but while closing the wound after the exploration it is timely and welcome.

I had a disabled patient who had no conscious memory of his surgery, but in hypnotic regression heard his neurosurgeon say during back surgery "I'll fix him" (Thing 10), and he never recovered from surgery. All I did in trance, after learning the surgeon's comment, was reword it to "I'll repair this." Along with a normal neurological exam and reassurance that his MRI and x-rays were OK, he went into a work hardening program and returned to work after two years of barely getting out of a chair.

82. Adrenalin (epinephrine) fixes memories

This is so true that Weinberger et al. (1984) were able to do Pavlovian conditioning of rats under general anesthesia by injecting epinephrine at the time of a sound and electric shock stimulus.

In the waking state subjects showed aversive behavior on hearing the sound, while controls that were injected with saline did not.

Fear is our most powerful emotion, and trauma releases adrenalin. The instinct for self-preservation leads us to imprint dangerous memories and be alert to avoid similar incidents. Post-traumatic stress disorder is the strongest imprint of all.

83. No need for rapport in an emergency

No need for rapport in an emergency, just credentials. We all know the imperative need for rapport when doing psychotherapy. This need disappears in an acute emergency situation, and hypnotic techniques are effective even when used by a complete stranger. The first law of nature is self-preservation, and when there is an explosion, rape, dislocated shoulder, baby crowning, and so on, the patient's mind is focused on fear and survival, and a hypnoidal state occurs. Fear overrides all logic and the victim turns to anyone with believable credentials for help.

My only induction with these patients is "I'm Dr. Ewin, I can help you. Will you do what I say?" With a "yes" answer to that, I can say "Fine, you're safe now. Close your eyes, take a deep breath, and turn this over to me. You can let your thoughts and feelings go off to your laughing place while I do what's necessary to get you well." I ask for an ideomotor signal when they find the "laughing place," and then I can relocate a dislocated shoulder, suture a laceration, or set a fracture. Since the patient's comfort is the issue, not proving how great hypnosis is, I don't hesitate to add some local anesthetic if it's handy.

James Esdaile recognized this principle when doing surgery in India in 1850. He wrote "In subjecting my patients to the sanative influence of Mesmerism for bodily complaints, no mental rapport has ever been thought of. ... In the management of mental disease, it will probably be required" (Esdaile 1850).

84. Easiest suggestion is "Keep doing what you're doing now."

It seems logical that as the autonomic nervous system is controlling body functions, it surely knows what it is doing right now. Our bad ideas come without effort and our good ones should come the same way. If what is happening is desirable, then a suggestion to keep doing what you're doing right now should be easy to accept without effort.

With acutely burned patients the standard initial emergency room protocol is to give a shot of analgesic and cover the burned area with iced towels. So by the time I get to the ER the analgesic is taking effect, the burned area is iced, and all I need to say is "Notice how all the involved area is cool and comfortable. When you are aware of this, signal by raising this finger (I touch an index finger)." When I get that signal, I say "Fine, keep it that way until it's healed."

I had a colleague who did acupuncture for pain. He told me he had several patients with reflex sympathetic dystrophy who would get pain relief from acupuncture lasting for twelve to forty-eight hours, and then have recurrence of pain. Studies have shown that acupuncture relieves pain by releasing encephalins (natural opiates), and is inhibited by the opiate antagonist naloxone. Hypnotic pain relief uses a different path and is not inhibited by naloxone. We treated five patients who had undergone six weekly acupuncture treatments with only temporary relief. While they were pain free, I did hypnosis with a suggestion to "Notice how comfortable it feels, and that your body can keep it that way." Three of them got complete relief in one combined treatment. One got more than 50 percent relief, and one was no better. My colleague has moved to another city and university, and we have not continued the experiment.

85. Best suggestions are ten words or less

Even though we're treating people with words, we talk too much in trance. After I've done my explaining in the waking state, and given suggestions in trance, it helps to summarize the message into about ten words or less, and repeat it three times or more to make it stick. For instance when I give Levitan's pre-op suggestion (Thing 54), I summarize "Less than helpful – Chinese," and repeat it at least three times.

Historically, the very inclusive self-hypnosis suggestion of Emile Coué (1905) resulted in many remarkable cures. He had patients repeat twenty times, twice daily, "Every day, in every way, I'm getting better and better." Ten words.

Good political slogans are short and repeated often. I can still recall from high school history sixty years ago that "Tippecanoe and Tyler too" helped elect William Henry Harrison as our ninth president. "I like Ike" did it for Eisenhower, and "Yes, we can" worked for Obama. A suggestion should stick in the mind like a slogan.

When I first saw Monet's *Impression, Sunrise* (the painting that gave its name to the impressionist movement in art), I realized that even though one could write pages about the scene with its colors, focus, contrasts, and so on, just the two words in the title sufficed to fix it all in my memory.

86. ETKTM
(Every Test Known To Man)

An ETKTM comes for hypnosis as a last resort. He/she has seen numerous specialists and been through at least one prestigious clinic, had every test known to man (except one), and has been told that all the tests are normal and basically there's nothing wrong with you. But the question remains, "Why do I keep having headaches, feel tired all the time, cry easily, forget things, sleep poorly, and (a list of other disorders of the nervous system)?" When I started listening to these patients in depth, I realized that in general most of them were what I call "normally neurotic." They weren't nuts. There was something wrong with their health. I found it in Hans Selye's research on 15,000 lab animals. He called it the General Adaptation Syndrome (Selye 1946), describing the physiological changes that occur with *chronic stress* of any kind.

The chronically stressed individual goes through three stages: alarm, resistance, and exhaustion. Chronic stress exhausts the adrenal cortex and the thymus (immune T-cells), and patients get functional hypoglycemia and autoimmune disorders. The entire nervous system is supplied with diminished fuel (glucose) and malfunctions. The test that *wasn't* done is a five hour glucose tolerance test (GTT). The Hypoglycemia Support Foundation http://www.hypoglycemia.org has a useful questionnaire that I use to prompt me to order a five hour GTT if the score is over 20. Note that the usual three hour GTT is useless for making this diagnosis, as is a single blood sugar determination at the time of the worst symptoms. When the blood sugar drops more than 20 mg/dl below the fasting level on the five hour GTT, the test is positive and warrants a trial of diet change. The patient needs to be on a six feeding, low refined sugar, low refined starch, and no alcohol or caffeine diet, along with hypnosis for relief of the chronic stress (Thing 75).

87. "Don't let your failures go to your head" – William Kroger, MD

This is an amusing way to give good advice to new students of hypnosis. Too often a novice is unsure of the technique, communicates this to the patient (Thing 78), gets a poor result, and then abandons hypnosis.

When I did my first induction, as soon as I got eye closure I opened the book and read the script to the patient. It worked, and very soon I could say it in my own words without reading. Accepting the fear of failure inhibits initiative and is picked up by the patient (Things 27 and 78).

Tom Edison said that in his lab he'd never had an experiment that failed, but he'd learned ninety-nine things that don't work.

88. Burns have two parts

It is not widely recognized that a burn has two separate components – the external heat injury to the skin and the internal inflammatory response to the injury (Thing 31). Anyone who has been sunburned knows that when leaving the sun there is some pain, but the heat injury is over. Then after several hours the blisters, fever, pain, and swelling occur. The initial *pain* is the body's alarm system saying "do something, there's danger," but the subsequent *pain* is inflammatory (the cardinal signs of inflammation are calor, *dolor*, rubor, and tumor (heat, *pain*, redness, and swelling)). Initial pain is transitory, inflammation is long lasting. The bradykinins (enzymes) that induce inflammation are released in the first two hours, and if the patient can be hypnotized in those two hours (even the first four hours), and can hallucinate that the involved area is "cool and comfortable," it cannot also be hot and painful, and no inflammatory enzymes are released. When the inflammatory part of a burn is thus aborted, the burn does not progress from first to second degree, or second to third degree, and there is minimal pain during healing.

Just as one can have the external burn stimulus with no response, one can have an internal inflammatory response without a physical stimulus. Using a cold coin on the patient's forearm, Dr. Chertok's film (1982) shows a blister developing after he suggests "It will cause a blister, as though it were hot."

The Indian firewalkers go through a week of fasting, sexual abstinence, and mental preparation ritual, then dedicate the firewalk to the Gods. Occidentals who participate in this (hypnoidal) ritual can do it too. The Fiji firewalkers believe that the volcano goddess gave their tribe a gift of being immune from being burned. They need no ritual.

89. Surgical analogy

I like the analogy of hypnosis to surgery. If a person has appendicitis, we start with an anesthetic. This facilitates the surgery, but does not cure. Recover from the anesthetic without surgery and the patient still has appendicitis.

Trance induction works like the anesthetic – it facilitates treatment, but if there is only induction and alerting, the patient is still sick.

In surgery, it's the operation that cures the patient. But it has to be the *right* operation – an appendectomy. A cholecystectomy or hysterectomy won't do it.

In hypnosis, it's the suggestion that cures, but it must be the *right* suggestion.

Our analytical skills lead us to find the right suggestion. In surgery, the patient still has to finish healing. If he gets an appendiceal stump abscess and it ruptures, he's no better off than if he'd never had an operation.

In hypnosis, the patient has to accept the suggestion or he will not improve.

Inductions are easy. Our workshops are to learn how to sort out the *right* suggestion and how to make it *acceptable* to the patient.

90. Informed consent for surgery

Informed consent for surgery may stir the pot of the Law of Pessimistic Interpretation (Thing 63). In my state of Louisiana, in an attempt to protect surgeons from a rash of malpractice suits claiming failure of informed consent, the legislature passed a law stating that a patient who signed a standard consent form had been fully informed. The standard consent said "I understand and acknowledge that the following known risks, among others, are sometimes associated with this procedure and/or anesthesia: brain damage, disfiguring scars, paralysis, including quadriplegia and paraplegia, the loss of or loss of function of body organs, and the loss of or loss of function of any arm or leg." This has since changed, but at the time it was a horror story that a patient should not read alone. If there are known specific common complications of a procedure, I write this down and review it individually.

Regarding the old standard form, I didn't want my patient having right brain visions of any of the noted horrors happening, and kept the discussion in the left brain. I'd first say to the patient "You surely know that there is some danger to any major anesthetic and surgical procedure, don't you?" "Yes." "Well, the law says that I must inform you of the worst things that can happen to people in the course of major surgery, and get you to sign this form saying that we have discussed it. There have been cases where someone died, was paralyzed, lost a limb, etc. Any questions? Sign here." I don't want my patient drifting into a hypnoidal state and daydreaming any of this happening to him (Thing 63). In his mind, I want these to be things that happen to other people!

I saw a patient for treatment of a reflex sympathetic dystrophy of his left lower extremity. He had ruptured the left Achilles tendon and had a good tendon repair, but the skin scar was adherent to the tendon and movement was limited. His orthopedist referred him to a plastic surgeon to release the scar, a relatively simple procedure. The nurse handed him the above release to sign, and he read it carefully, including the clause about losing use of a limb. He signed it, said nothing, underwent the procedure, and post-op lost use of the limb. When I saw him he was on crutches with no weight bearing.

We know that all suggestion is self-suggestion
(Things 62, Law 5, and 63).

91. We experience emotions in our bodies

Frustration often leads to a headache, the betrayed person feels he's been stabbed in the back, controlled anger causes a knot in the stomach, and a startle makes a heart skip a beat.

Psychosomatic medicine is best practiced when we can change the idea that evokes the symptom. The target organ identifies itself.

92. Tapes and self-hypnosis

Many of my confreres report excellent results teaching patients self-hypnosis. I must not do it right, because I have not been able to replicate their success enough to be highly enthusiastic about it. However, I do use self-hypnosis for myself regularly.

Since our bad ideas come without effort, I believe that our good ideas should come the same way, and listening to a tape is effortless. I make a tape with a short induction, appropriate suggestions, and an alerting set, and do the same for myself as for my patients.

93. Post-hypnotic triad

When a deep trance subject is given a post-hypnotic suggestion, three things happen:

i. Compulsive carrying out of the suggestion.

ii. Verbal amnesia (source amnesia) for the origin of the idea.

iii. Rationalization of the behavior.

This meshes with what happens when a patient has a fixed idea (Janet's *idée fixe*), and particularly when the fixed idea leads to a phobia. The idea can be resisted, but only at the expense of an anxiety attack. A person who is phobic about an elevator can force himself to get into it, but he is in a cold sweat, pulse racing, blood pressure up, and tense. He will gladly climb ten flights of stairs to avoid the anxiety attack. He cannot explain why he feels this way (source amnesia). When asked why he climbs the stairs, he may rationalize by saying that he does it for exercise.

94. The duty of the subconscious mind is to protect the organism

The first law of nature is self-preservation. Any creature that does not protect itself becomes extinct.

The subconscious functions to make it automatic, reflexive, and intuitive to take self-protective positions at all times. Symptoms are often irrational attempts at safety – see constant pain (Thing 32) and adrenalin fixes memories (Thing 82).

95. Response to cortisone or antihistamines

Response to cortisone or antihistamines often gives a hint that a medical disorder is also amenable to hypnosis.

Asthma, hives, and most of the autoimmune disorders respond to hypnosis approximately as well as they do to cortisone, without the dangerous side effects.

96. Hypnotizability is not an issue with ideomotor signaling

Ideomotor just means an idea is activating a motor movement. This is a form of body language and all people normally have body language in the waking state. Both highs and lows unconsciously nod their heads when saying "Yes" and shake their heads as they say "No."

In trance, it is much easier to exert the minimal effort of finger signals than to do head shaking, but either will work.

97. Direct Suggestion in Hypnosis (DSIH) and hypnoanalysis

Direct Suggestion in Hypnosis (DSIH) and hypnoanalysis are as different as night and day. We teach *DSIH* in our basic workshops and have large books of scripts to use for different situations. Hypnotizability is a major issue in success with this technique, and in my experience it gets little better than a placebo response, maybe 50 percent (only 20 to 40 percent for smoking cessation). DSIH is better than a placebo because it seals an idea, and doesn't wear off like a placebo.

Hypnoanalysis, using ideomotor signals, gets closer to 80 percent results and hypnotizability is not an issue. It can be done in the waking state with a pendulum. It is insight therapy and identifies the dystonic idea, allowing replacement (reframing) with a syntonic idea. When a hurtful idea has been changed to a healthy one, a long term cure is accomplished.

I would rather treat a low hypnotizable patient by hypnoanalysis than a high by DSIH. Graham and Evans' research (1977) shows that highs treated with DSIH relapse more frequently than lows.

98. Closed eye roll induction

The Hypnotic Induction Profile (HIP) is a rapid test of hypnotizability, and it includes an open eye roll. Many clinicians use it as an initial induction to assess what kind of response they are likely to get using direct suggestions.

I have found that when a patient has a low score on the eye roll it lowers my expectation of success, it dampens my enthusiasm, and it hurts our rapport. So I decided that I don't want to know a patient's hypnotizability before starting treatment – it can always be tested later since it is a stable trait.

I have my patient close his/her eyelids first, then roll the eyeballs up and take a deep breath (my usual induction), avoiding a readable eye roll sign. Since hypnotizability is not an issue when using my preferred technique of hypnoanalysis (Things 96 and 97), I believe that my clinical outcomes have been enhanced rather than diminished by not testing initially.

99. I want to talk

When doing hypnoanalysis with ideomotor signals, an important signal to set up is "If something crosses your mind that you want to tell me, or you want to ask a question, just raise your hand (extend patient's wrist) and we'll talk."

A patient will not ordinarily *initiate* speech while in trance (Thing 57), but has no problem with a motor signal. Much significant free association goes on during trance, and the time to access it is while it is occurring, not at debriefing. In fact, much of it is lost once the patient is alerted and back into left brain processing.

100. Spirituality

Spirituality is very different from religiosity. One does not need to belong to any organized denomination or sect to wonder about the meaning of one's own life. It is psychologically depressing to lead a meaningless life, and many of my depressed patients have lost track of the idea that *all* of our Creator's children are *precious,* even though none are perfect (Thing 14). We are responsible for making our own lives meaningful, useful, and joyful, and when a patient feels his life is meaningless, I consider it a spiritual problem.

Nobody goes to the doctor to get his religion changed, and I don't preach to my patients, but just saying that my perception is that the patient has a spiritual problem seems to open doors and cause a different kind of introspection that is often productive. Rather than the Bible, a quote from the Declaration of Independence is a good starting point: "We hold these truths to be self-evident, that all men are created equal, that they are endowed by their Creator with certain unalienable rights, that among these are the right to life, liberty, and the pursuit of happiness."

101. Post-Concussion Syndrome

Post-Concussion Syndrome is worth mentioning because in my experience it is most often the result of poor communication and error in diagnosis, and therefore of iatrogenic (physician generated) origin. Anatomically, the cerebrum is the *brain*, and a true *cerebral concussion* is a *temporary* physiological (not neurological and no MRI abnormality) dysfunction of the brain, followed by full recovery (as occurs when the leg "falls asleep" during a movie). It includes being unconscious and losing short term memory of the accident. This differs from a *cerebral contusion* which causes clear injury to the brain, with neurological and MRI changes, and may have long term consequences.

Pliny the Elder said "He who saw the lightning and heard the thunder is not the one who was struck." So when a patient who had a blow to the scalp (remember the brain is protected by a bony skull) tells me all the details of the accident, I know he wasn't *brain* injured even if he believes he was momentarily unconscious. The correct diagnosis is a *scalp contusion*, and that's like a contusion to the arm, leg, or any other part of the body that happens in any football game. The scalp is sore for a while, and gets well.

The word "concussion" has meaning to lay persons very different from what I have written above. When a doctor tells a patient he had a concussion, without pointing out that his neurological exam is perfectly normal and his prognosis is excellent (whether he thinks he was unconscious or not), a bag of worms is opened up. He goes home and tells his wife that the doctor said he had a concussion, she tells her friends, there are questions about any headaches or behavior changes (nocebos, Thing 54), and so on, and when the doctor sees the patient next week he's full of subjective symptoms that are not explainable on a physical basis, and disability may have set in already. There are exceptions to this, but in head injuries we must be particularly careful what we say.

Mittenberg et al. (1992) showed that "Imaginary concussion reliably showed expectations in controls of a coherent cluster of symptoms virtually identical to the post-concussion syndrome reported by patients with head trauma."

References

Baglivi, G. (1704). *The Practice of Physick Reduced to the Ancient Way of Observations.* Cited by J. P McGovern and J. A. Knight in *Allergy and Human Emotions* (1967). Charles C. Thomas, Springfield, IL.

Beecher, H. K. (1956). Evidence for increased effectiveness of placebos with increased stress. *American Journal of Physiology* 187: 163–169.

British Thoracic Society (1983). Comparison of four methods of smoking withdrawal in patients with smoking related diseases. *British Medical Journal* 286: 595–597.

Cheek, D. (1959). Unconscious perception of meaningful sounds during surgical anaesthesia as revealed under hypnosis. *American Journal of Clinical Hypnosis* 1: 101–103.

Chertok, L. (1982). *Can Your Mind Control Your body?* BBC documentary.

Colloca, L., Sigaudo, M., and Benedetti, F. (2008). The role of learning in nocebo and placebo effects. *Pain* 136: 211–218.

Coué, E. (1905). Article/essay title?. In R. L. Charpentier, *L'Autosuggestion et son application pratique.* Les Editions des Champs-Elysées, Paris.

Cousins, N. (1979). *The Anatomy of An Illness As Perceived by the Patient.* W.W. Norton, New York.

Esdaile, J. (1850). *Mesmerism in India.* Longman, London. (Repr. as *Hypnosis in Medicine and Surgery.* Julian Press, New York, 1957.)

Ewin, D. M. (1977) Hypnosis to control the smoking habit. *Journal of Occupational Medicine* 19: 696–697.

Ewin, D. M. (1980). Constant pain syndrome: Its psychological meaning and cure using hypnoanalysis. In W. J. Wain (ed.), *Clinical Hypnosis in Medicine.* Year Book Publishers, Chicago and London.

Ewin, D. M. (1983). Emergency room hypnosis for the burned patient. *American Journal of Clinical Hypnosis* 26: 5–8.

Ewin, D. M. (1987). Constant pain syndrome: Its psychological meaning and cure using hypnoanalysis. *Hypnos* XIV: 16–21.

Ewin, D. M. (1989). Letters from patients: Delayed response to hypnosis? *American Journal of Clinical Hypnosis* 32: 142–143.

Ewin, D. M. (1990). Hypnotic technique to recover sounds heard under anesthesia. In B. Bonke, W. Fitch, and K. Millar (eds.), *Memory and Awareness in Anaesthesia.* Swets & Zeitlinger, Amsterdam.

Ewin, D. M. (1992). Hypnotherapy for warts (verruca vulgaris):41 consecutive cases with 33 cures. *American Journal of Clinical Hypnosis* 35: 1–10.

Ewin, D. M. (1994). Many memories retrieved with hypnosis are accurate. *American Journal of Clinical Hypnosis* 36: 174–175.

Ewin, D. M. (1998). Editorial comment on Felt et al. *American Journal of Clinical Hypnosis.* 41(2): 138.

Ewin, D. M. and Eimer, B. N. (2006). *Ideomotor Signals for Rapid Hypnoanalysis: A How-to Manual.* Charles C. Thomas, Springfield, IL.

Evans, F.J, (1989). Presented at the 40th annual meeting of the Society for Clinical and Experimental Hypnosis.

Felt, B. L., Hall, H., Olness, K., Schmidt, W., Kohen, D., Berman, B. D., Broffman, G., Coury, D., French, G., Dattner, A., and Young, M. H. (1998). Wart regression in children: Comparison of relaxation-imagery to topical treatment and equal time interventions. *American Journal of Clinical Hypnosis* 41: 130–138.

Freud, S. (1900) *The Interpretation of Dreams*. In the *Standard Edition of the Complete Works of Sigmund Freud*, vols. 4 and 5, ed. and tr. James Streachey. London, Hogarth, 1953.

Graham, C. & Evans, F. J. (1977). Hypnotizability and the deployment of waking attention. Journal of Abnormal Psychology, 86: 631-638.

Heath,G.H. (1996). *Exploring the Mind-Brain Relationship*. Moran Printing, Inc., Baton Rouge,Louisiana.

Heart of Healing (1992). *What You Become*. Noetic Sciences documentary aired on TBS stations.

Holy Bible. All quotes in the text are from the King James Version.

Kline, M. V. (1958). *Freud and Hypnosis*. Julian Press, New York.

Kluft, R.P. (2007). A Pragmatic Approach to Risk Reduction in the Clinic and the Workshop. Presented at the 59th Annual Meeting of the Society for Clinical & Experimental Hypnosis. Anaheim, California, October 24.

Levinson, B. (1990). The states of awareness in anaesthesia in 1965. In B. Bonke, W. Fitch, and K. Millar (eds.), *Memory and Awareness in Anaesthesia*. Swets & Zeitlinger, Amsterdam.

Mason, A. A. (1952). A case of congenital ichthyosiform erythrodermia of Brocq treated by hypnosis. *British Medical Journal* 23: 422–423.

Mason, A. A. (2007). Presentation at the annual meeting of the Society for Clinical and Experimental Hypnosis, October 27, Anaheim, CA.

Mittenberg, W., DiGiulio, D. V., Perrin, S., and Bass, A. E. (1992). Symptoms following mild head trauma: Expectation as aetiology. *Journal of Neurology, Neurosurgery, and Psychiatry* 55: 200–204.

Orne, M. (1982). *Hypnosis on Trial*. BBC documentary film.

Osler, W. (1905). *Aequanimitas: With other addresses to medical students, nurses, and practitioners of medicine*. P. Blakiston's Sons, Philadelphia, PA.

Peacock, S.M. (1954). Physiological responses to subcortical stimulation. In *Studies in Schizophrenia*. Heath, R.G. (Ed), The Tulane University Department of Psychiatry and Neurology, pp 235-248. Harvard University Press, Cambridge, Massachusetts

Pedersen, D. L. (1994). *Cameral Analysis: A Method of Treating the Psychoneuroses Using Hypnosis*. Routledge, London.

Rossi, E. L. (1991). *The 20 Minute Break: Using the New Science of Ultradian Rhythms*. Jeremy P. Tarcher, Los Angeles, CA.

Sarbin, T.R. (2006). Hypnosis as a conversation: 'believed-in imaginings' revisited. Contemporary Hypnosis 14 (4): 203-215

Selye, H. (1946). The general adaptation syndrome and the diseases of adaptation. *Journal of Clinical Endocrinology* 6: 117–230.

Servan-Schreiber, D. (2004): *The Instinct to Heal*. Rodale Press, Emmaus, PA.

Service, R. (1940). *Collected Poems of Robert Service*. Dodd, Mead & Co., New York.

Tindle, H. A., Rigotti, N. A., Davis, R. B., Barbeau, E. M., Kawachi, I., and Shiffman, S. (2006). Cessation amongst smokers of "light" cigarettes: Results from the 2,000 national health interview survey. *American Journal of Public Health* 96: 1498–1504.

Weinberger, N., Gold, P., and Sternberg, D. (1984). Epinephrine enables Pavlovian fear conditioning under anesthesia. *Science* 223: 605–607.

Weitzenhofer, A. (1957). *General Techniques of Hypnotism*. Grune & Stratton, New York.

Praise for
101 things I wish I'd known
when I started using hypnosis

I have often described the remarkable Dr. Dabney Ewin as "a treasure". Now in *101 Things I Wish I'd Known When I Started Using Hypnosis*, he has given the hypnosis world a treasure chest full of the gems and pearls he has polished in his 40 years of practicing medical hypnosis. Dr. Ewin describes hypnosis as "an empathetic involvement with another and as we interact with our patients/clients we evolve in our tone of voice, choice of words, what we emphasize, and our timing". This cogent, concise resource is a gift of shared wisdom from an evolved master to assist the next generations of clinicians in mastering the art of hypnosis. "101 Things" helps the novice as well as the accomplished clinician learn what to say, when to say it and how to say it. Dr. Ewin often remarks that "we are all created precious" and this little gem certainly is precious.

Linda Thomson, PhD, APRN, ABMH

In general conversation, Dabney M. Ewin, M.D., is a congenial, meticulously courteous Southern gentleman, a pleasant and unfailingly interesting companion. However, when conversation turns to the clinical use of hypnosis, without Dabney's manifesting any apparent change in his appearance, behavior or demeanor, one's experience of Dabney undergoes a metamorphosis. One rapidly appreciates that he or she is in the presence of an unusual and gifted clinician, for whom the term "therapeutic genius" is a pallid understatement. In fact, the more knowledgeable one is about hypnosis, the more easy it is to appreciate that Dabney Ewin is so skilled that he stands as an almost mythical figure in the world of hypnosis, conjuring up associations to Merlin, Gandalf, Yoda, and, more recently, Albus Dumbledore. As my experience grows in depth and in breadth, I continue to find in Dabney an inexhaustible fund of skill and wisdom. A few years ago my son was burned in an accident. I was given an upsetting estimate of his injuries. As I drove to the hospital I utilized some of Dabney's techniques over the telephone. When I arrived, the physician attending to my son apologized for having overestimating the severity of the burn wounds! My son healed without either scars or disfigurement, thanks to a skill I had learned from Dabney Ewin. In *101 Things I Wish I'd Known When I Started Using Hypnosis*, the reader encounters Dabney Ewin reflecting on many topics and offering insights into what he has learned along the way in his distinguished career. 101 Things… is a pathway into the experience of learning from Dabney Ewin. This is a book to read slowly and reflect upon, observation after observation. It will not serve as a textbook or a "good read." For those readers who have had the pleasure of knowing and/or learning from Dabney, it offers a chance to review and reflect, with many a smile, on the many (and still-evolving) facets of his approach to helping the hurt, the ill, and the suffering. For those readers who have not yet had the good fortune to know and learn from Dabney, I am confident that this introduction to him and his approaches will incline many of them to make their way to his workshops.

Richard P. Kluft, MD, PhD, President, Society for Clinical and Experimental Hypnosis, Past President, American Society of Clinical Hypnosis

The first thing that struck me about this book was the title – *101 things I wish I'd known when I started using hypnosis*. As a seasoned practitioner and teacher of hypnotherapy I asked myself 'how needed is a snapshot of an experienced and respected practitioner's innermost thoughts and feelings into his work with clients?'. The answer was 'desperately'!

On further reading, his initial explanation of the idiosyncrasies of our definitions of what our clients need to be 'doing' both excited me and called into mind the term 'Thank you!'. What a relief to see an author make what may be a commonsense differential statement between words such as 'stop' and 'quit', which at first sight may not mean much when working with clients, until you realise that they may understand the power of language, but on many occasions do not resonate with its importance for them.

This insightful exploration into the complexities of language continues into much sought after areas of knowledge that both practitioners and clients desire, including working with pain and many other common complaints.

This is a short book, but do not let that mislead you as to its importance. I am reminded of Yalom's Gift of Therapy, when I say that some 'short' books are career definers. This is up there with the best of them in terms of succinct, wise, inspired insight, and I recommend it for any therapist who either needs to know more, or who needs some fire in their belly to reignite their love of therapy.

Tom Barber MA, Course Director,
Contemporary College of Therapeutic Studies

For a small book it carries a big punch!

This is definitely a 'must have' for anyone who uses hypnosis in their work or in their practice. For therapists, doctors, social workers, teachers and nurses - it has something for everyone, no matter how experienced you may be.

Dr Ewin has written a very practical, no-nonsense, down to earth book based on his own experiences and is passing on some real pearls of wisdom within its pages. He isn't sharing with you a new theory on hypnosis, but instead allows you to find your own way to use these 'pearls' within the framework that you already use. To him, patient/client power is key to the healing process and this is obvious throughout the book.

Whether you are an 'old hand' or just learning, this book really should be part of your library.

Terri Bodell FNACHP, Deputy Chair,
National Association of Counsellors, Hypnotherapists and Psychotherapists

In a world where attention to words, the use of metaphors, and assisting people to be relieved of pain and suffering all intersect, we are in the land of hypnosis. Beyond the research labs and clinician's office, the inhabitants of this world teach each other through their shared experiences, their anecdotes and stories, modeling the wise nuggets as they teach. Dr. Ewin, affectionately known as Dabney, has compiled 101 nuggets of hypnosis wisdom from decades of practicing medicine. He would call them pearls of wisdom, but pure gold better captures both their value and the effort it takes to gather them. The result of our courage, our ignorance, sometimes our hubris, and almost always our mistakes, wisdom is hard won, especially when our goal is to help others. How do we know what psychological ingredients are right for patient X? Dabney reminds us, we often do not know, but if we trust our clients' subconscious, it knows and with hypnosis we can help our clients access what they need to heal.

The preface of the book sets the tone with Dabney's down home style and his ever-present modeling of the use of hypnotic language and metaphors. He tells us "Read the little book" a suggestion you will feel compelled to follow. He has utilized the KISS principle (Keep it simple, stupid) with expertise and tongue-in-cheek humor. With unusual candor and warmth, again modeling, the trust he shows the reader builds rapport quickly. We feel safe reading his 101 pieces of advice- To the hypnotically initiated these are familiar pitfalls. Dabney observes them without judgment, only encouragement for us to learn. We can identify with each anecdote with which he illustrates his accumulated knowledge. How many of us, indeed, in those early days of learning, read the scripts while the patient's eyes were closed? Dabney dares to share his learning process and thus invites us into the hypnosis community where suggestions are both explicit and implicit. He has us watch as he does "rounds". By item number 54, I could hear him saying, 'this patient taught me…' and I realized that more than enthusiasm, the essence of his contribution is the reverence and respect for his patients. He wants them to get better and has shared a lifetime of reflections on what has helped him to help others hypnotically. We can all benefit from these reflections.

Dabney is an outstanding educator and a lifetime learner. Reading 101 things I wish I had known when I started hypnosis, one realizes there are always more things to be learned. The book's design is a simple prescription: meditate on one item a day.   And pay special attention to item number 38 which reminds us that a patient's name carries emotion. Acknowledging that item and all the linguistic spandex I have nurtured in my hypnosis training, I heartily recommend this book and know that " a little Dabney'll do you".

Julie H. Linden, PhD, Past President, American Society of Clinical Hypnosis and President-Elect of The International Society of Hypnosis

This little book is going to be an invaluable resource for practitioners of both hypnotherapy and psychotherapy, drawing, as it does, on the long experience of the author and his acute observations which have obviously stood him in good stead during his career.

The book is full of common sense advice on avoiding the pitfalls many therapists (and medical practitioners) are apt to fall into. Simply by avoiding the use of words which may have negative connotations for clients or patients and substituting words which will be less likely to be viewed pessimistically, therapy can be even more successful and a speedier outcome can be reached. Even pronunciation can have its unforeseen problems. The author cites a case where he lost rapport in an instant with an English client simply by using the Irish pronunciation of her name (Kathleen) at a time when the IRA bombings were rife in the UK.

Dr. Ewin believes absolutely in the power of the mind/body connection and recommends that therapists undergo many of the hypnotic techniques themselves, since it is so much easier to be confident about a procedure if it has already been successful for oneself. He also advocates the use of humour in healing – something that many newly qualified therapists tend to steer clear of, believing that helping people to resolve their problems should be a 'serious' undertaking.

I have to say that I agreed wholeheartedly with Dr. Ewin's approach, finding nothing in the book about which I could say "Oh, I wouldn't do that!". In fact, his methodology put me very much in mind of the late, great, Duncan McColl, from whom many therapists in this country learned so much during the last twenty or so years.

In short, I would recommend this book to anyone who wants to learn in a very short space of time what most therapists only learn from years of experience.

Pat Doohan, Fellow of the National Council of Psychotherapists and also of the International Council of Psychotherapists. (FNCP & FICP), Editor of Fidelity, the in house publication of the NCP/ICP.

About the author

Dabney M. Ewin, MD, FACS, ABMH is a board certified surgeon and occupational medical specialist. Early in his career he was plant physician for the Kaiser Aluminum plant in New Orleans, and started using hypnosis for some badly burned patients. He became interested in psychosomatic medicine, developed a private hypnosis practice, and began teaching hypnosis at Tulane University Medical School in 1970, and at Louisiana State University Medical School in 1980.

Dr. Ewin is a life member of the American Medical Association, Fellow of the American College of Surgeons, and former speaker of the House of Delegates of the American College of Occupational and Environmental Medicine. He is a past president of both the American Society of Clinical Hypnosis (ASCH) and the American Board of Medical Hypnosis. He is a Fellow and past secretary of the Society for Clinical and Experimental Hypnosis (SCEH) and a member of the International Society of Hypnosis (ISH). He has received the Milton Erickson Award of ASCH, the Roy Dorcas Award of SCEH, and the Pierre Janet Award of ISH. He has published numerous articles on hypnosis and is co-author of the book *Ideomotor Signals for Rapid Hypnoanalysis: A How-to Manual*.

He serves as Clinical Professor of Surgery and Psychiatry at Tulane University Medical School and Clinical Professor of Psychiatry at Louisiana State University Medical School.